Chakra Healing For Beginners

I0413898

How To Unblock Your Chakras

For More Health, Love, Wealth & Creativity

By Hester Waite

The following book is reproduced below with the goal of providing information that is as accurate and as reliable as possible. Regardless, purchasing this book can be seen as consent to the fact that both the publisher and the author of this book are in no way experts on the topics discussed within,

If you like my book, please leave a positive review on Amazon. I would appreciate it a lot. Thanks!

BONUS IN THE BACK:

Take a look at my other books too. These are the titles:

NLP For Beginners

Parenting For Beginners

Contents:

Introduction

Congratulations on purchasing your personal copy of *Chakra Healing For Beginners.* Thank you for doing so.

The following chapters will discuss some of the many ways that your chakras work for you and how you can clear them out for optimal use.

You will discover how important it is to keep your chakras working at the best so that you feel your best. Knowing how to open and clear your chakras is important, but it can also seem daunting. With the right guidance and some awareness, you can clear your chakras and feel better than you ever thought possible.

In this book you will discover:

- What chakras are

- The affect that all seven of them have on your body

- Positive energy and vibration

- How to clear your chakras

- Chakra meditation

- And much more

You will discover that opening your chakras aren't as hard as many people think. It's something that you can achieve, and it can be done by implementing some of the practices that this book provides. Get this book and get started today.

The final chapter will give you some chakra meditation practices that you can start using today.

There are plenty of books on this subject on the market, thanks again for choosing this one! Every effort was made to ensure it is full of as much useful information as possible. Please enjoy!

Chapter 1:What Are Chakras?

The word chakra is a Sanskrit term which means disk or wheel. When the word is used in Ayurveda, yoga, and meditation, it is referring to the wheels that move the energy through the body. Within the body, seven chakras help to align the spine beginning at the base of the spine, and traveling up to the top of the head. When you visualize a chakra, visualize a wheel of swirling energy where your consciousness and matter connect. This is known as Prana, an invisible energy. It is important to live and keeps us alive, vibrant, and healthy.

Each of these swirling energy wheels matches up with your body's massive nerve centers. They each contain a group of major organs and nerves and controls your spiritual, psychological, and emotional well-being. Since everything in the world and your body is moving, it's important that your seven chakras are fluid, open, and aligned. If you have a blockage, your energy isn't able to flow. Look at a chakra like a drain in your bathtub. If you let your hair gather at the drain, the water is going to start to backup, stagnate, and then mold and bacteria will start to grow. This goes for your chakras as well. Fixing a bathtub is simple, it's physical.

Keeping your chakras open is a bit harder, but not as hard when you have awoken your awareness. It's important to become aware of imbalances in different areas of your life because spirit, soul, body, and mind are so closely connected, and once you notice the imbalance, all the other areas will come into balance.

Let's look at an example. Think of a woman who has just lost her husband. She ends up getting sick, developing acute bronchitis. The illness stays in her chest, and she ends up have pains in her chest each time she coughs. The entire heart chakra is affected by this. If she can realize that her loss and bronchitis is connected, she will be able to heal a lot faster once she begins to honor the grieving process. She has to treat the grieving along with the physical ailment.

Matter Chakras

Your first three chakras, all located close to the base of the spine, are known as chakras of matter. They tend to be more physical in nature.

The First Chakra – Muladhara, The Root Chakra

This chakra is located at the base of your spine, the first three spinal vertebrae, and the pelvic floor. Muladhara can be broken down into two Sanskrit words: Mula, which means root, and Adhara, meaning base or support.

Having a balanced root chakra gives you a good, solid foundation for opening all your other chakras. This is the foundation that your house is built upon. This chakra is made up of all the things that keep you stable in life: safety, shelter, essential water, food, and emotional needs. When all of these needs are met, you feel more balanced and safe.

When this chakra is imbalanced, you may experience nightmares, anxiety disorders, or fears. Physical problems can come up as issues with the feet, leg, lower back, bladder, and colon. Men can experience prostate problems. Eating disorders can be connected to root chakra imbalance.

The Second Chakra – Svadhisthana, The Sacral Chakra

This chakra is found right above the pubic bone and just below the navel, and surrounds the hypogastric plexus and genital area. Svadhisthana is translated to the dwelling place of the self. The element associated with the second chakra is water, which represents cohesiveness.

When your second chakra is balanced, you will feel joy, pleasure, abundance, and wellness. When it isn't balanced, a person can experience addictions, depression, sexual dysfunction, fear of change, and emotional instability.

The Third Chakra – Manipura, The Solar Plexus Chakra

Manipura means lustrous gem. This chakra is located around the bellybutton and solar plexus area all the way to the bottom of the breastbone. This chakra provides you with the power to transform, warrior energy, self-esteem, and personal power. It also has control over your digestion and metabolism.

You know that your third chakra is open when you feel self-motivated, have a sense of purpose, and are self-confident.

Spirit and Matter Connection

The Fourth Chakra – Anahata, The Heart Chakra

This chakra is the center of all the chakras, with three above and three below. This is where the spiritual and physical meet. It is located in the middle of the chest, and also covers the breasts, lungs, thymus gland, cardiac plexus, and heart. Anahata means unhurt or unstruck. This chakras name implies that below grievances and pain of the past there is a spiritual and pure place where there isn't any hurt.

When your fourth chakra is open you have lots of compassion and love, you accept yourself and others, and forgive easily. When your heart chakra is closed, you will feel hatred to others and yourself, fear of betrayal, jealousy, anger, and grief.

Spirit Chakras

The Fifth Chakra – Vishuddha, The Throat Chakra

This is the first spiritual chakra. It controls the areas of the larynx, tongue, mouth, neck, jaw, parathyroid, and thyroid. When your throat chakra is aligned and open you will be able to express yourself, listen, and speak from a higher place. Understanding and faith are the essences of this chakra.

The Sixth Chakra – Ajna, The Third Eye Chakra

This chakra is located between your eyebrows. It encircles the lower area of the brain, head, eyes, and pituitary gland. This is where your intuition sits. Ajna means beyond wisdom. This will lead you to spiritual knowledge that can lead you if you allow it to. When your sixth chakra is open, you will experience visualization, expanded imagination, lucid dreaming, telepathy, and clairvoyance.

The Seventh Chakra – Sahaswara, The Crown Chakra

This chakra is also known as the thousand-petal lotus. This is the last chakra and located at the top of your head. This is where you spiritual and enlightened connection comes from. It's what connects you with your higher self, to all the other beings on earth, and the divine energy that made all celestial beings.

When this chakra is open, you have become pure awareness. You are expansive, undivided, and pure consciousness. Just like a raindrop in the ocean, you are only a part of the ocean that holds and encircles all of it.

Since this book is about opening and clearing your chakras, it's important to understand the key aspect of balancing your chakras. This key element is awareness. The human body is always fighting between imbalance and balance. Unless there is a clear problem in a particular area of your body, it can be quite hard to figure out where your imbalance lies. This is why it is so important for you to be aware of your body.

Chapter 2: Positive Energy and Vibrations

Many people go through life without knowing that their thoughts and mind shape their world. The thing is, though, the quality, polarity, and nature of your thoughts are profoundly intertwined with your reality. Your physical and mental move together, they walk hand in hand. From several different angles, you can see why meditation, and your chakras, significantly affect you positive energy and vibration.

Everything is the universe is some form of energy. You may be able to see it, or you can feel it, you navigate through several different types of energy as you go through your day. Whether it's negative, positive, or neutral, you create energy. Everything you do, everything you say, everything you do not do, and everything you think emits their types of vibration that are sent out into the universe.

If begin focusing your actions, thoughts, and words so that you create more positive energy, you will notice your life improving in amazing ways that you didn't know that you could. All things in your life, and everyone you cross paths with a start to move to a higher vibrational plane.

Think of how amazing it would be if you could transform into a positive beacon of energy. With everything you do, and everywhere you go, you spread a beautiful light. You use your higher vibration to make the world just a little bit better. You can do this through meditation, and clear your chakras.

When you meditate, you create this conscious shift, which makes you more aware of the highest truth, we are all just one. Rich or poor, atheist or religious, republican or democrat, or black or white, we are one, united. Humans are more alike than different. Everybody has the basic needs, motivations, and wants: love, purpose, happiness, and health.

Through meditation, you are reminded of these things. When you become able to see your face in other, something amazing happens: everyone is now your other-self. They are only you in a different timeline and another form.

In the law of attraction belief system, your ideas and thoughts send out vibrations to the cosmos. Then the universe responds to these vibrations and sends back a customized set of experiences which validates the things you believe and thought.

Because your thought becomes your life, you are the creator of your circumstances. For instance, if your mind is constantly filled with limiting beliefs, such as "I'm not going to get the promotion… I'm never going to find happiness… I'm never going to be good enough" guess what? You're not going to be. You're not going to be those things because those feelings tell the universe what you should experience.

The tricky thing is, the universe doesn't discern between don't want and want. Everything is sent to you that you ask for. So the key thing so to remove your self-imposed limited beliefs.

The next thing is to let go of resistance. Picture life as a river your canoeing on. Do you want to paddle against the current, taking ten times longer, and wasting ten times more energy? Or do you want to paddle with the current, allowing it to move you along to your destination gently?

Whether you realize it or not, it is most likely, you are living your life against the current. People try hard to control everything that happens to them; they don't see the purpose of the hard times. They resist circumstances, and thoughts will become negative and toxic when things don't go the way they want.

This is another aspect that meditation can help with. The deep thought that is achieved during meditation helps you to understand the polarity of the universe. If there weren't any bad, then there wouldn't be any good. There has to be opposition in all things. This is essential to being able to experience life to its fullest.

Now, think of your body as a cobweb auric field. It traps all different types of energy, especially the negative energy.

Eventually, you become weighed down with fear, stress, and worry. This is where clearing out your chakras come in handy. This is typically done during meditation. You will be able to tap into the quantum source which is in everything and everyone. I will tell you more about this later in the book.

Chapter 3: Chakras and Abundance

There is probably a level of frustration constantly living in you if you are stuck living paycheck to paycheck. The attachment of "not having enough" tends to be so strong that it causes people to live in fear, act on impulse, and become stressed. Think that over. How many of your family or friends do you know that completely loathe their jobs, yet they stay with them because they are worried they won't be able to get another?

If you find that you are having problems obtaining and maintaining abundance in your life, chances are your root chakra is blocked. The root chakra connects you with the physical world. This is where we receive the tools to wealth. Remember, wealth does not always mean money. True abundance is what is within you. You do have to figure out how to access this abundance. While, the last chapter of this book is full of meditations to help balance your chakras, and the chapter before talks about clearing chakra, I am going to go over some ways to attract abundance into your life through your first chakra.

Meditation can connect you with a higher spiritual plane; it also works to ground you. You may find it hard to trust that the world is going to provide you with what you need to survive, but when you're connected to a higher self and trust a higher power, you will have what you need to feel safe.

It doesn't matter if you refer to this higher being as Spirit, God, Mother Nature, Source or Consciousness. When you are connected to a universal energy, you have a sense of stability and peace. Wild animals are not sure if they will be able to find food from day to day, yet they can trust that nature will provide.

Do this: Your sense of smell is connected to the root chakra. When you meditate, try focusing on the tip of the nose to align you root and to call upon the thing you need to balance the root chakra.

Let's look at five steps you can take to bring more abundance into your life:

1. Figure out where you have discomfort

Are you afraid of going for your dreams because you may not achieve what you have thought up? Do you hate going to work? When you dig deep, you will realize which emotions and thoughts could be causing your success to be snuffed out. Nurture any anxiety and fear you may have by accepting where you currently are and make the conscious decision to make what you want coming true.

2. Let go of the things that aren't working for you

After you have figured out what is holding you back, it is time to let it go. Take a piece of paper and write out your worry. Begin the statement with "Dear... (write your discomfort), thank you for the concern, but I don't need you any longer. I have learned from you to trust who I am and the process that (your higher belief) has planned for me. I would like for you to leave in peace and continue to send me blessings." Then, all you have to do is release it. This can be done by tearing it up or burning it, whatever symbolism works best for you.

3. Come up with a security plan

So you have figured out your problem, and you have let it go, now you need to come up with a success plan. The first chakra likes structure, so when you come up with a success plan, you will also be waking up your root chakra. Write everything that you want to have in the order you wish to attain it. Make sure you affirm the desires in the now. This means, instead of saying, "I want to attract my dream job," say "I am fully capable of attracting my dream job. Success has surrounded me!" Make sure you are practical and that you set goals realistically. Think about where you want to be in one, three, and six months.

4. Energize the root chakra

Once you have your success plan written, you have to give it energy. Fold your plan four times. As you do so, affirm what you want to attain and thank your higher being for helping you in this process. Once you have folded your paper, hold the plan at the base of the spine and visualize a red light coming from it. Notice the heat from the light moving from your hand to your root and start thinking about how amazing it feels to make you dreams real.

5. Keep going

The last thing to do is take action. You have to do work to catch up with your abundance. Unfortunately, some people think that their desires are going to miraculous appear in front of them. There have been some amazing miracles happening, maybe, but action is the most important component of turning your dreams into reality. Start paying attention to inspired thought. You know inspired thought because it will pop up out of nowhere. This could mean a person, place, or your divine source. It is pretty much a cosmic aha moment. Please DO NOT second guess yourself. If it feels right, then do it.

The more often you work with your first chakra; you will start to see more measurable changes. The most important thing you can do to make sure you create you abundant life is to stop focusing on money and focus on making abundance. There is a huge amount of abundance to go around. Money just comes and goes. The power is in you to use it. You have a lot more abundance than you think.

Gems, Colors, Sounds, and Asanas

There are many ways to open up your root chakra, which includes gems, colors, mantras, and yoga.

The most effective yoga asanas for Muladhara are:

- Malasana, squatting pose

- Padmasana, lotus flexion

- Janu Sirsansana, head to knee pose

- Pavanamuktasana, knee to chest pose

Kegel exercises can also help women to awaken their root chakra, and women and men can practice Bandha Yoga. This helps to bring strength and energy to the region of your root chakra.

Toning sounds and chanting can also bring balance to your first chakra, just like music is able to bring people together. Sounds will cause a vibration in your body, and these vibrations allow the cells to work in harmony. LAM is the mantra sound that works with the root chakra.

Gems and colors can also be used to balance your root chakra. Red is the corresponding color for the root chakra. Bloodstone, black tourmaline, red jasper, and garnet are the gemstones associated with your first chakra. You can open and align the chakra by placing one of these gemstones on your root chakra while laying down.

Chapter 4: Chakras and Creativity

Creativity is part of human nature. You can express this creativity through procreation, but the power of the second chakra isn't limited to creating babies. You create when you garden, cook, or bake. When you figure out a solution to a problem, you are creating. Whenever you have raw materials, mental or physical, and turn them into something, you use your creative energy.

The sad thing is, our creativity tends to be discouraged, especially with education. After we make it through the phase of life where cutting paper, coloring, and painting is acceptable, society expects us to mold into non-creative beings. For us to conform, we tend to lose creative energy, and, in the process, our unique ideas. As adults, we quickly become used to following the latest trends, what others find acceptable, and what is right. Then, if we are asked to think abstractly, we may find it quite difficult.

In certain areas of your life, you may feel creative and open, but in others, you feel self-conscious. For instance, you may feel completely comfortable with painting a beautiful picture, but when asked to write an essay or cook a meal with a recipe, you might not feel as comfortable. The important thing to do is rise to the occasion and take the risk.

The main reason why people stop taking creative risks is that, at some point, somebody has told them they weren't good at something. To be able to open your second chakra, you have to be willing to take the risk and not worry about failure.

Playing is a great way to start this. Think of how a child plays. Children will spend hours building a sandcastle, a block tower, or dollhouse. Then, a second later, they are willing to smash it to bits and start over.

Start playing like those children. If the dinner you spent hours cooking does not turn out right, who cares? If your new plant dies a week after you planted it, plant a new one. If a project at work flops, it does not mean that your whole career is over. Just a like a child playing, begin again. There is an infinite amount of energy inside of you just waiting for you to tap into it.

Not only does being open to creativity help to balance your sacral chakra, but having a healthy sex life, respecting, and honoring your body helps as well. Start getting in touch with your feelings and see if there are any old emotions that you are hanging onto. Start working through those feelings in a healthy way.

Ida Nadi, left nostril breathing, helps to open your sacral chakra because it brings in fourth lunar energy. With your first two fingers on your right hand, close your right nostril and breathe in and out through your left nostril eight to ten times.

Gems, Colors, Sounds, and Asanas

The following asanas can help to open your second chakra:

- Cobra pose, Bhujangasana

- Butterfly pose with forwarding fold, Baddha konasana

- Seated pelvic circles

The VAM mantra sound can help to awaken the second chakra. Orange is the associated color for the second chakra, and hematite, carnelian, calcite orange, and amber are its gemstones.

Chapter 5: Chakras and Digestion

With clear intentions, goals, and desires, you are able to move towards achieving them. Every little step you take while working to honor your big intention will help you to strengthen your solar plexus chakra. The Sanskrit word Tejas means the fire within and is the fire found in the Ayurvedic dosha Pitta. When a person has a strong Pitta, they have the inner drive needed to move them toward their goals.

It doesn't matter what your dominant dosha is, you are still able to harness your third chakra power so that you can assert your will in a way that is healthy and will help you to achieve your goals. If you have a decision that you are stuck on or you're at a crossroads in life, look to feelings in your gut to help guide you.

1. Begin by closing your eyes, place a hand on the part of your belly just above the navel.

2. Start thinking about the dilemma or problem.

3. Take note of how your third chakra feels when you give it different choices regarding your problem. If you feel nauseated or receive a sinking feeling, then that decision is wrong.

4. If you give your solar plexus a good option, you will feel lightness or may even be able to breathe better.

Agni, digestive fire, is also housed in this chakra. To make sure that your third chakra stays open, you need to make sure that your digestive fire stays healthy. To keep a powerful Agni, follow these guidelines:

- Allow the stomach to rest between meals. When you graze or snack frequently, your body doesn't have the time to replenish Agni. It can only do this if the stomach is resting.

- Take little drinks of water when you eat and do not drink fruit juice, soda, and alcohol. When you drink too much while eating your digestive acids will become diluted, but when you drink alcohol, you produce excess acid.

- If you are a Pitta dosha, avoid spicy foods.

- To keep from overeating, eat around two cupped handfuls at each meal.

- Avoid adding ice to beverages, drink them slightly warm or at room temp.

Gems, Colors, Sounds, and Asanas

With yoga, any pose that causes heat to develop in the solar plexus is great for stimulating your third chakra. This includes boat pose (Navasana), seated spinal twist (Matsyandrasana), and warrior.

RAM is the mantra sound associated with the third chakra. Chanting this can help you to open your chakra.

The associated color is gold or yellow, so any gemstone in one of these colors can open your solar plexus and bring more energy to the stomach, pancreas, liver, and spleen. Tiger-eye, golden yellow labradorite, and yellow topaz are great gemstones to have for your third chakra.

Chapter 6: Chakras and Love/Relationships

Some people choose to live in areas of grievances. They have probably been hurt in the past by lovers, classmates, friends, siblings, or parents. You may have been in one of those positions as well. It is pretty much impossible to stay away from those situations where you may be hurt by somebody. It is up to you to decide what to do with that hurt. Some may choose to hurt the person that hurt them. That is not living with an open heart chakra. A person who is willing to inflict pain on somebody else is coming from hatred, fear, or ignorance, all of which manifest with a closed heart chakra.

Whenever you experience hurt from your past or present, you have the choice of fully experiencing them and letting them go, or holding onto them. When you let them go, you can open your heart to new things with understanding, compassion, and love. When you hold onto the hurt, you will start harboring negative feelings, and it will end up cutting you off from things you love. Allowing yourself to let go is as simple as making a choice. Your ego and mind will tell you otherwise, but it is as simple as making that decision.

Being able to put yourself in another person's shoes is no easy feat, but it can help you to feel empathy. An excellent way to learn compassion and empathy is to play something called "the what if scenarios." Whenever you encounter somebody that has been unpleasant towards you or has treated you badly, start going through a list of what ifs. Some examples would be, "What if they received bad news?" "What if they are having a bad day?" "What if they just lost their job?" "What if somebody in their life was diagnosed with an illness" or "What if they found out their spouse was having an affair?" When you start building these endless stories, you will start to empathize with the person and their situation. This will remove you from self-pity and make you feel compassion for the other.

Let's look at the fact that there may be a friend or family member that repeats this pattern of inflicting hurt constantly. You should still offer them compassion and love either by creating boundaries or from a distance. Just remember that whenever somebody decided to hurt you, it is pretty much never about you, it is them.

To ensure that you get love is to give love. Leo Buscaglia, a motivational speaker and author, taught that people need to receive and give 12 hugs each day for good health. Some other ways to bring love in are:

- Go at least one day a week without criticizing anybody, and this includes you

- Give co-workers, friends, and family positive feedback and affirmations

- Forgive and forget. There is no sense in holding grudges

- Smile at everybody you see, even though you may not feel like smiling

Take any chance that you can to spread love around, and you will feel better too.

Gems, Colors, Sounds, and Asanas

When performing yoga, practice poses that brings heat into the heart chakra. Some of the best poses are cow face, standing bow, and camel.

YUM is the mantra sound associated with the heart chakra. If you want, you can use this special mantra to open your fourth chakra, OM MANI PADMA HUM. When you repeat this during meditation, you will increase your heart chakra powers.

Emerald green is the associated color. The best gemstones are rose quartz, jade, malachite, and emerald.

Chapter 7: Chakras and Voice

True expression is not something that comes easily. There is a fragile dance between saying what you mean and being diplomatic or tactful. It is easier to say what the other person wants to hear instead of telling the truth. Judgment from others or fear of being rejected could keep you from telling the truth.

Working on your lower chakras will prepare you for this kind of communication. When you get the first two chakras aligned, it will help you overcome your fears. Opening the third chakra will give you a feeling of personal power, and you will have the confidence of expressing yourself. If you know what is in your heart, this came when you align the fourth chakra. When you need to verbalize your opinions, desires, and needs, you will be able to know how to be truthful to others and yourself.

If you are used to accommodating others, instead of saying what you would like to say, you might have to practice out loud. Affirmations are used when you want to make your desires reality. Write down what you want to say to others. For example, what if you want to ask your boss if you can work from home a few days each week, but you just don't have the courage to ask him? Write down what you want to say and practice saying it in front of a mirror.

You might like it if your in-laws would learn to call before they come over but you don't like confrontation. Write down this request, practice it, a lot, and include some responses they might say back to your request.

Listen and speak with compassion. There are three gateways that you have to cross before you speak:

1. Ask yourself if what you are going to say is true.
2. If it is, go to the next gateway and ask if what you are about to say is absolutely necessary.
3. If this answer is yes, go to the next gateway and ask yourself if what you are going to say is kind.

Speaking truthfully does not mean that you can be critical or hurtful. The truth from the spiritual essence will be compassionate and kind.

Listening is another feature of the fifth chakra. The best way to listen is to give the other person your full undivided attention. This means you need to put away your electronic devices or turn them off when others are speaking. You need to learn to wait to hear the other completely before you respond. We have, after all, two ears and just one mouth, so we can listen twice as much as what should come out of our mouths.

Gems, Colors, Sounds, and Asanas

Reading, humming, singing, and chanting aloud are great ways to open this chakra. The mantra sound for the fifth chakra is HUM. Two Pranayama exercises that stimulate and heat the throat chakra are the Ujjayi breath and the lion's breath.

You can do the plow or Halasana, shoulder stand or Salambe Sarvangasana, bridge pose or Setu Bandha Saragasana, and camel pose or Ustrasana. These will stimulate the parathyroid and thyroid glands and bring the energy to the throat area.

The color that corresponds with this chakra is blue. Gems that can balance this chakra are turquoise, aquamarine, lapis lazuli, blue topaz, and sapphire.

Chapter 8: Chakras and Intuition

The world is experienced with the five senses. Before you passed through your mother's womb, you heard noises such as your mother's heartbeat and voice. You also heard muffled sounds outside. You experienced light, taste, and touch. Since your moment of birth, you have attributed your experiences to what you get through your senses. You have learned to trust your senses in what you hear, see, touch, smell, and taste. While sense perception is wonderful in life's experiences, it does limit you when you want to expand your awareness.

There was a time when you had to count on a sense of inner knowing and intuition. We all had to rely on signals we got from the environment and even primal instincts to guide us before we had modern technology. Birds can sense when bad weather might hit, squirrels know when they need to gather food for winter, we humans have an intuitive sense as well. We have lost touch with it and our ability to trust it.

Our physical senses can give us clues as to how to follow our intuition. Have you ever felt like your milk had gone bad? You check the expiration date, and it is still good. You smell it, and it feels fine. You ask someone else if the milk is still good. You haven't hit on anything concrete to tell you that the milk is bad, so you drink a glass. Shortly afterward you start experiencing bad stomach pains. This is because, on a subtle level, your sense of smell gave you a subtle clue that you doubted.

You are making a business deal with someone, and everything looks great. The person seems to be honest and great. When you shake hands with them, you feel like something isn't right. When the deal is done, you find out it was a corrupt deal.

You get these clues through senses, but when something seems off, you have a tendency just to ignore it. There is good news. You can learn to trust these clues and make good decisions based on your senses. When your decisions are right, write them down to reinforce the fact that your intuition guided you in the correct decision. Just like the animals in the forest, you have always had a sixth sense. You just need to find it and follow it.

You can use your inner sense for guidance to help you make the right decisions. Take into account your ego, intellect, mind, and your soul in making decisions. Just like you turn to your solar plexus to guide you with discomfort or comfort, you pay attention to that subtle feeling or hunch as to whether you need to go forward or hold back. If you feel conflicted, ask your intuition to open itself up to you so you can make the correct choice.

Just like all the other chakras, Ajna is balanced with meditation. People who are new to meditating report having a tingling feeling at the third eye or think it is just a headache. A pulsating or tingling sensation around the third eye either after or during meditation shows that you are opening your third eye.

A great breathing technique or Pranayama is called the bee breath or Brahmari. Bring both of your hands to your face. Put the two middle fingers over the eyes. Let the index fingers rest on the eyebrows and the pinkies under the cheekbones. Stop up your ears with your thumbs. Take a deep breath and exhale with the work AUM with an emphasis on the M sound while making a buzzing sound like a bee does. Do this for two minutes. You will alleviate tension in your head, and it will help open the sixth chakra.

Gems, Colors, Sounds, and Asanas

Any yoga or Asana pose where the forehead is pressed down is good for the sixth chakra. Try the child's pose or Balasana with your forehead pressed on the yoga block or the floor. Dolphin's pose is another pose where you lift the head up and look toward the floor.

The sixth chakra's color is indigo, and the mantra sound is SHAM.

Gems that will help to open the Ajna chakra are azurite, lapis lazuli, and amethyst.

Chapter 9: Chakras and The Divine

The lotus flower is used by both the Buddhist and Hindu traditions. It gets nurtured, grows, and emerges from muddy waters. It will bloom where you will find no clarity. The lotus's beauty is unique to its environment that is monotonous and does not have any vibrancy.

When you get to the opening of the seventh chakra, you will emerge through confines of your physical body, your ego, mind, and intellect. You will push beyond the soul that ties you to Samsara which is the endless cycle of birth and rebirth. You will be freed from desire's shackles. White light will surround your body, and you will appear to stand out from the murky surroundings.

When you read the description of the seventh chakra, it might look like it is out of reach. You might think that sounds great for gurus and monks but not for you. You are just ordinary and have a normal life.

We have demands of our daily lives, and our busy minds accompany these demands. Attaining enlightenment might not be so far off. A good goal might be to live in a state of awareness. Try living with moments of pure awareness. All of us have experienced moments like this one time or another. Have you ever felt an overwhelming love for another? Have you experienced a miracle?

Practicing daily silence, prayer, and meditation are disciplines that will lead to increased moments of spiritual connection. These are the only way you can experience the very essence of Sahaswara. You go to school hours every day to study for exams and to get a degree. Silence, prayer, and meditation are the studies you need to get a spiritual degree.

When you have figured out your daily practice schedule to do these activities that will connect you to your universal consciousness, you will see your spiritual awareness expand into your outer world. You will start to have unconditional love consistently. You will become more forgiving, kind, and compassionate. You will show more humility. Life will not be just about you and what you want. Your life will be more about serving other people because when you serve others, you are in turn serving yourself.

Gems, Colors, Sounds, and Asanas

While silence is the most important and powerful way to open the seventh chakra, other practices can support this chakra.

Two Pranayama breathing techniques that you can do before beginning meditations are Nadi Shodhana or alternate nostril breathing and Kapalabhate, or the shining skull breath.

Inverted yoga asanas like the headstand or Salamba Sirsasana and downward facing dog or Adho Mukha Svanasana could help to stimulate the seventh chakra. Any posture that will bring the crown of your head to the floor like a fish pose or Matsyasana. Other poses that can help are the corpse pose or Savasana, this would be best done on the ground or grass, and the half lotus or Ardha Padmasana is a good meditation pose.

Using essential oils during prayer, meditation or massages can help to awaken the Sahaswara. These oils have some physical effects, too. They can help provide muscle relief, migraines, and headaches. These oils include:

- Spikenard helps with emotional balance and promotes restful sleep.

- Lavender helps provide peace and calmness.

- Rose Oil: this oil has the highest spiritual frequency. It is used for harmony, transformation, and spiritual insight.

- Lotus: this is a general oil that can be used for emotional and spiritual ailments.

- Helichrysum: is used to get through deep psychological barriers.

- Vetiver: this oil is used to stabilize and calm.

- Sandalwood: is used the quiet the mind.

- Frankincense: this is a holy oil that is used for meditative contemplation.

The color for this chakra is white, or violet and the mantra sounds like the universal sound OM. Gems you could wear or have within your environment to help you to open and align this chakra are sugilite, selenite, and amethyst.

Chapter 10: Clearing Your Chakras

If you have stiffness or achiness or certain fears and emotions, it would help to find out which chakra is blocked or affected.

Root or First Chakra

Physical imbalances in this chakra could include problems with the prostate gland, male reproduction system, immune system, tailbone, rectum, feet, and legs. Those who are suffering from a physical imbalance have a higher chance to experience issues of constipation, eating disorders, sciatica, knee pain, and degenerative arthritis.

Emotional imbalances might include feeling that affects our survival needs like the ability to provide for life's necessities, food, shelter, and money.

When this is in balance, you will feel supported. You will feel as though you are safer and more unified with the world around you. You will feel grounded.

The lesson of this chakra is self-preservation. We have the right to be here.

Sacral or Second Chakra

Physical imbalances with this chakra could include reproductive and sexual issues, low back pain, pelvic pain, hip, kidney dysfunctions, and urinary problems.

Emotional imbalance might include being about to commit to relationships. We have problems expressing our emotions. We can't have fun, be creative, experience pleasure, play based on desires, or express sexuality. You will note this one through fear of addictions, and impotence.

If this chakra is in balance, we will be able to take risks. We are committed. We are creative. We are outgoing, sexual, and passionate.

This chakra's lesson is to honor others.

Solar Plexus or Third Chakra

If this chakra is out of balance, you might have physical imbalance of colon diseases, gallbladder and pancreas issues, stomach ulcers, diabetes, high blood pressure, chronic fatigue, liver dysfunction, and digestive problems.

Emotional imbalances can include issues with our inner critic comes out, self-esteem, and personal power. We will fear of physical appearances, criticism, and rejection.

If this chakra happens to be in balance, we will feel far nicer towards ourselves. We will feel confident, assertive, and in control.

This chakra's lesson is self-acceptance.

Heart or Fourth Chakra

If this chakra is not balanced, you could have physical imbalances of wrist or arm pain, shoulder problems, upper back problems, lymphatic systems, issues with breasts, lung disease, heart disease, and asthma.

Emotional imbalances will include bitterness, anger, abandonment, jealousy, issues of the heart, and over-loving to almost suffocating others. You will have a fear of loneliness.

If this chakra is balanced, we will feel compassion, love, gratitude, and joy. Forgiveness will flow freely, and trust is gained.

This chakra's lesson is I Love.

Throat or Fifth Chakra

Physical imbalances with this chakra might include shoulder and neck pain, problems with the tongue, lips, cheek, chin, ulcers, ear infections, TMJ, laryngitis, sore throats, and thyroid issues.

Emotional imbalances will include problems with self-expression by communicating either written or spoken. Fear of not having any power or choice, feeling out of control or no willpower.

If this chakra is balanced, we will have free flowing communication, expression, and words. We are truthful and honest but firm. We will be good listeners.

This chakra's lesson is let your voice be heard.

Third Eye or Sixth Chakra

If this chakra is imbalanced, you might have physical problems like hormone function, hearing loss, seizures, eyestrain, sinus issues, blurred vision, and headaches.

Emotional problems might include problems with self-reflection, volatility, and moodiness. We cannot look at our fears, and we do not learn from others. We catch ourselves daydreaming a lot and live in our own internal imagination.

If this chakra is in balance, then we are focused, clear, and we can tell the difference between illusion and truth. We become open to getting insight.

This chakra's lesson is seeing the big picture.

Crown or Seventh Chakra

If this chakra is out of balance, we will have problems with environment, sound, light sensitivity, learning inability, and depression.

Emotional imbalances will include problems with greater power and self-knowledge. These imbalances come from an overactive mind when it comes to spirituality and the world around us, worrying often and finding ourselves prejudiced. We have a very deep-set worry of being annoyed.

If this chakra is in balance, we will find it far easier to live moment-to-moment. We have an unshakeable trust of our inner guidance.

This chakra's lesson is to live mindfully.

You might feel like you have more than one chakra out of balance or blocked. This happens when one is blocked, the others try to compensate and become under or over active.

The easiest way to balance them is to start at the bottom and work your way to the top.

You can rid yourself of dormant energy by cleansing your chakras.

Our energy has to constantly be in a state of flux, so that they don't get stopped up – when they get stopped up, less than pleasurable side effects appear.

However, when you get rid of the energy that has become stuck, you can heal different conditions, regardless of what plane of reality they are on.

The schedule by which you rid yourself of dormant chakras is up to you. You can do it every time that you meditate, as a way of just keeping the pipes clean, or you can do it to free some dormant energy to fix any problem that you might be facing.

If you are wondering how exactly you will benefit from getting rid of dormant energy, I will just say that there are a ton of ways.

Allow me to list a few:

- Been depressed lately? Cleanse the chakras to make you feel uplifted and lighter.
- Nauseous as of late? Get the chakras in your solar plexus moving again.
- Head pounding? Sounds like your third eye could use some care – cleanse it.

- Having a sudden pimple breakout? Acne is the way that dormant energy shows itself. Cleanse the chakras and heal those blemishes.

It is incredibly simple and fast to learn the proper way to cleanse chakra and release stagnant energy.

Here is a way to cleanse your chakras:

1. Grounding Meditation: For every practice regarding intuition, making sure that you are grounded is the very first thing you will need to do. You will use the Earth's energy that you get from the grounding meditation to run through all of your chakras. This step is critical.

2. Open Chakras: When you have finished the grounding meditation, begin with the root chakra and open each chakra one by one. This is easily done. All you do is imagine each one opening. I like to think about a rose opening for each of the chakras. Give each one a certain color:

   a. Root Chakra: Red

   b. Sacral Chakra: Orange

c. Solar Plexus Chakra: Yellow

d. Heart Chakra: Green

e. Throat Chakra: Blue

f. Third Eye Chakra: Purple

g. Crown Chakra: White

Beginning with the root chakra, think about a rosebud sitting at the bottom of your spinal cord. Visualize it blooming blissfully. When it has bloomed completely, you know that the root chakra has opened and that you can go to the next chakra. Try to visualize every single bud growing into a full bloom as you make your way up to the top of your head. Some might like to use different colors of doors opening, or maybe a combination of different things. After completing the grounding meditation, to get all the chakras should take about four to six minutes.

3. Send some energy through every chakra: Let's return to the grounding meditation. Do you remember the light which you brought forth from the Earth? Now let's take it a bit further. Start at the root and then visualize that

the energy is coming out of the root chakra. Think of it as an open faucet, through which liters of white energy are bursting and through that root chakra. Now, bring another string of white energy through the sacral chakra. Think about it as rushing energy through the sacral chakra. Now continue with this process until you have seven different strings of white energy flowing through every one of the seven chakras.

4. Turn the flow off: There is no definite way to end this. There is no set duration for which this has to last. Just allow your energy to be released until you're satisfied. The amount of time depends on each person and how much energy is needed to clear each chakra. It might take 5 minutes or 20. It is up to you to decide when it is the time for you to stop. Trust that whatever length of time you decide, it is the right time for you.

When that time is finished, start with the crown and pull out the energy streams like you are unplugging an appliance. One by one, think about them falling back to the Earth.

5. Close Chakras: When you have stopped the flow of energy, it is time to start closing each one. It is important to know that you are not shutting them completely, just partially. Having the chakras open completely is not sustainable for anyone at any time. With your chakras open completely, you run the risk of draining your energy. The Earth's energy has been turned off, and you are running on your energy. You run the risk of others noticing your generous giving state and take advantage of it. We do not want these things to happen, so we need to turn down the energy for each chakra.

Just like turning off the energy flow, we begin at the crown and think about a radio knob for each chakra. Think about turning the dial down to a point where you feel comfortable. If you get it too low, you might start to feel heavy, or anxious all of a sudden. Think about turning the dial to the right state for you. As you travel down the chakra highway, adjust the volume for each chakra, to a place that feels comfortable. This process is intuitive, and there isn't any right or wrong way it can be done. There is no too open or too closed. Every person has their state of balance. This point is different for every person.

Don't understand what feels right?

That is perfectly fine. Just pay attention to how you feel and what you physically experience when you open chakras, as you run the energy, and as you turn the dials. You are learning to be aware of subtle energy, and it will take time. Just practice – open, close, adjust until it feels right and you want to stop. With time, you will get the hang of it and be able to do this complete process in 15 minutes or less.

6. Clean up: Think about all the junk you just emptied out of your chakras piled around you. Now, take a broom and sweep all that chakra clogging junk into the garbage until it has all been cleaned.

You are done. Follow these steps any time you need to a quick, simple and effective way to clean your chakras.

Cleanse your chakras. Clear those pipes and allow pure, clean energy to flow freely. Allow yourself to feel energetically and physically healthy.

Chapter 11: Chakra Meditation

If the cause is not addressed, you will continue to feel distressed or upset in the emotions, mind, and body.

What causes the suffering and distress?

Suffering results when we believe we are separate instead of whole.

Basic identification is what creates our belief system. If we think we are a separate entity, our beliefs will be incomplete and inadequate. Our beliefs make our bodies, emotions, and thoughts.

When we start to experience that we are One with all that is, our lives, body experience, emotions, thoughts, our beliefs, we start to reflect the peace that we know we can be.

For a chakra meditation that allows the chakras to balance and heal themselves, do any meditations that can bring the attention to you as Pure Awareness. As we begin to focus on our Light, we release the things that stand in our way of feeling well and experiencing love.

During the time of getting to know our bodies as Pure Awareness, there are different meditations that we can use to identify us being separate rather that the whole that we are. Focus on meditation that works from the outside in.

For help with easing the effects of beliefs that may be painful, there are several versions of the light that you can include. Below are some examples:

- Diamond White Light will align and purify your energy field.

- Emerald Green Flame will transform and restore our bodies.

- Violet Flame combines the gold flame of Christ's Consciousness, the pink ray of the Divine Feminine, and the blue ray of the Divine Masculine.

- Rose Pink Light will infuse your being with the Love of Divine Mother and will create a protection bubble around and in you. This is great for protection and inner child healing.

- Sunshine Yellow Ray arises in our awareness and is associated with Christ's Consciousness as our feminine and masculine poles begin to balance. This ray is infused with Divine Illumination and Wisdom.

- Gold Light is deeper that the Sunshine Yellow Ray. It pulls peace into your which is an energizing nectar that will nurture and stabilize your energy field. This is a great light to bring into yourself after you do energy work, for completion and balancing.

As you start chakra meditation, just remember that you are opening your awareness of yourself and this will increase the awareness of materials that have been growing under the surface for many years or perhaps lifetimes.

You might notice that there has been an increase in uncomfortable sensations and feelings. It is just actually the awareness of underlying energies that increases and not the actual energy.

Healing is gradual. There are pieces of beliefs that turn free layer by layer. There is no reason to go digging to see what they are. Just realize what irritates you during your daily life, and it will let you know what is available for you to heal. This will be your window of opportunity.

As you continue with chakra meditation, your healing will open up its way and when it is ready. As long as we dream the dream, on our body's level, the healing will continue layer by layer, as we begin to awaken fully.

Since oxygenation and breathing are vital to the energy system, chakra meditation is vital in the process of becoming whole.

Here is how to balance and activate each Chakra:

Root Chakra

1. With all meditations, sit in a comfortable position with back straight but not rigid. Close your eyes and start with deep belly breaths. A good way to know that you are doing this right is to lie down and breathe in through your nose. You will notice that when you inhale, your belly will fill first then the chest will follow. The best thing about lying down is that it can't be done wrong. Once you have a feel for it and practice some, you can sit up.

Breathe deeply through the nose without separating between the exhaling and inhaling. You will start to feel yourself relaxing. Continue this for five minutes and be aware of your body as you breathe. Focus on your breathing as it goes in and out. Allow the breathing to become deeper and rhythmic. You should feel yourself becoming more relaxed with each breath.

2. Now focus your attention on the first chakra in the body at the base of the spine.

   Imagine you are breathing in and out through this first chakra. The air is going all the way down to the base of the spine on the inhale and out through the nose on the exhale without any separation between breaths. On every exhale, see the energy in the first chakra grow stronger with the meditation. See the chakra as a fireball growing stronger and brighter with every exhalation. Let your consciousness move into the energy ball. Become one with the energy ball and feel yourself being drawn down into the earth.

3. When this happens, pay attention to how you are feeling mentally, emotionally, and physically. Notice what you are experiencing. Everyone will be different. Some have experienced visions of the earth or the earth's cycles, belonging to nature and Mother Earth, death, and birth. By meditating on this chakra, you will be getting in touch with different aspects of your nature and connecting with your relationship with the earth.

Do this for ten minutes or until you feel satisfied. When you are ready to return to the present, say this, "Each time I am in the relaxed state, I will learn to use my mind creatively and will be more aware of the energy blocks that keep me a prisoner so I can heal myself." Release the energy ball and the vision and count to five. You should feel refreshed, peaceful and relaxed as you come back to the room and open your eyes.

Sexual Center the Second Chakra

1. If you are just doing one chakra, follow the first step under the beginning chakra meditation, otherwise please continue.

2. Put your attention on the second chakra at the base of the spine.

   Envision that you are breathing in and out through this second chakra. The air goes down to your sexual organs on the inhale and out through the nose on the exhale with no separation between breaths. With each exhale, feel the energy in the second chakra getting stronger. See the chakra as an orange ball that is growing stronger and brighter with each exhale. Let your awareness move down to the energy ball. Become one with the ball and feel yourself starting to radiate out from the center of your body and then out into the environment. Feel the magic and wonder that radiates from the second chakra with the meditation.

3. While this is happening, pay attention to how you feel physically, mentally, and emotionally. Notice what you experience. This will be different for each person. Some might feel bursts of energy going up and down their spine or through the entire body. These are normal. Just, relax and enjoy them. Some might feel a warm current or vibrations going through their body. These sensations show an increased flow of energy within the body. Be aware of the changes you are experiencing. Observe them, do not influence them in any way. By meditation of this chakra, you will be getting in touch

with different areas of your sexuality and the creative process.

Do this for ten minutes or until you feel satisfied. When you are ready to return to the present, say this, "Each time I am in the relaxed state, I will learn to use my mind creatively and will be more aware of the energy blocks that keep me a prisoner so I can heal myself." Release the energy ball and the vision and count to five. You should feel refreshed, peaceful and relaxed as you come back to the room and open your eyes.

Solar Plexus the Third Chakra

This chakra allows you to surpass the conscious mind and all the concerns so you can experience selflessness that will allow you to have a deeper connection with others.

1. If you are just doing one chakra, follow the first step under the beginning chakra meditation, otherwise please continue.

2. Now focus on the third chakra in your body. Think about breathing in and out through this chakra. The air should go down to the third chakra on the inhale and up through the nose on the exhale with not separation between the breaths. With each exhale sense the energy in the third chakra getting stronger. With this chakra meditation, see a yellow ball growing stronger and brighter with each exhalation. Let your consciousness more into the energy ball. Become one with the energy ball and feel yourself start to radiate out from that center through the body and into the environment. You will start to feel like you are melting.

3. While this is happening to pay attention to how you are feeling mentally, emotionally, and physically. Notice what you are experiencing. It will be different for each person. You might feel like you have become fluid and watery as your consciousness radiates out from this center. You might also feel great empathy. This empathy is a product of contentment and trust. It will allow you to feel compassion for the suffering and pain

of others and yourself. Give yourself to these feelings and allow them to flow through you.

Do this for ten minutes or until you feel satisfied. When you are ready to return to the present, say this, "Each time I am in the relaxed state, I will learn to use my mind creatively and will be more aware of the energy blocks that keep me a prisoner so I can heal myself." Release the energy ball and the vision and count to five. You should feel refreshed, peaceful and relaxed as you come back to the room and open your eyes.

Heart the Fourth Chakra

1. If you are just doing one chakra, follow the first step under the beginning chakra meditation, otherwise please continue.

2. Focus your attention on the heart chakra. Think about breathing in and out through the fourth chakra. The air will go down to your heart on the inhale and up through

the nose on the exhale with no separation between breaths. With every exhale, sense the energy of the fourth chakra getting stronger. During this meditation visualize a green ball of light growing stronger and brighter with each exhalation. Let your consciousness move into the energy ball. Become one with the energy ball and fell yourself radiate out from that center through the body and into the environment.

3. Feel the transformation of love what radiates through the heart and into the other chakras. Notice how you feel mentally, emotionally, and physically. The more you are centered with the heart, the more you will feel the mystic heart in you and your consciousness. As the river of living water radiate through the heart, your body with begin to pulsate with energy from the top of your head to the bottom of your feet. Currents of energy will shoot everywhere. You will get warming pulses coming from your heart and fills the entire body. If you surrender to the energy that radiates through the heart, you will experience unconditional love and compassion

for everyone and yourself. You might also experience a feeling of peace that surpasses all understanding.

Do this for ten minutes or until you feel satisfied. When you are ready to return to the present, say this, "Each time I am in the relaxed state, I will learn to use my mind creatively and will be more aware of the energy blocks that keep me a prisoner so I can heal myself." Release the energy ball and the vision and count to five. You should feel refreshed, peaceful and relaxed as you come back to the room and open your eyes.

Throat the Fifth Chakra

1. If you are just doing one chakra, follow the first step under the beginning chakra meditation, otherwise please continue.

2. Focus your attention on the throat chakra meditation. Think about breathing in and out through the throat chakra. The air will go in and out your throat with no

separation between breaths. With each exhale, sense the energy in the throat chakra growing stronger. During the meditation, see a blue ball of light getting stronger and brighter with every exhalation. Let your consciousness move into the energy ball. Become one with the energy ball and feel yourself start to radiate out from the center through the body and into the environment.

3. Feel yourself become full of courage, noble and fearless. Experience the honesty of choosing yourself in each moment. Feel the inner affirmation that will say yes to every moment in life. By being centered in your throat, it allows you to feel more triumphant. You will experience victory in each moment without making anyone else feel small. You can repeat to yourself, "I am free at last" over and over again.

As you experience this, you might feel energy shooting up your spine. As it goes past the throat, it will become currents of unconditional joy. You will fulfill your purpose in life by accepting the victory.

Do this for ten minutes or until you feel satisfied. When you are ready to return to the present, say this, "Each time I am in the relaxed state, I will learn to use my mind creatively and will be more aware of the energy blocks that keep me a prisoner so I can heal myself." Release the energy ball and the vision and count to five. You should feel refreshed, peaceful and relaxed as you come back to the room and open your eyes.

Third Eye the Sixth Chakra

1. If you are just doing one chakra, follow the first step under the beginning chakra meditation, otherwise please continue.

2. Focus your attention on the sixth chakra. Think about breathing in and out through the third eye. The air will go in and out with no separation between breaths. With each exhalation, sense the energy in the third eye getting stronger. During this meditation, visualize an

indigo blue ball getting stronger and brighter with every exhale. Let your consciousness move into the ball of energy. Become on with the energy ball and feel yourself start to radiate out from the center through the body and into the environment.

3. Feel yourself becoming one with others. Feel your mind going in all directions and fill the room with your consciousness. Focus on how your feel mentally, emotionally, and physically. The more you can center your third eye; the more complete the union of your unconsciousness and consciousness will be. This will produce an electric current going through your body, and your head will glow with your third eye.

   Do this for ten minutes or until you feel satisfied. When you are ready to return to the present, say this, "Each time I am in the relaxed state, I will learn to use my mind creatively and will be more aware of the energy blocks that keep me a prisoner so I can heal myself." Release the energy ball and the vision and count to five. You should feel refreshed, peaceful and relaxed as you come back to the room and open your eyes.

How you experience the chakra meditation is what is right for you in your present moment. As you clear and heal your energetic system, the way you meditate will change, too. Never judge yourself. Allow yourself to grow at your own pace. Give yourself the gift of the fourth chakra to love yourself with unconditional love and compassion.

Crown or the Seventh Chakra

There isn't any meditation possible with the crown chakra since people can't exist as a separate being.

By meditating on each of the seven chakras, you are activating awareness of the emotional feelings and blocks. These come in various ways for different people. This depends on the gifts that you have developed already. Clearing and removing energy blocks will enhance your gifts by making you stronger or opening yourself up to new abilities that you were not aware of before. Whatever happens is perfect for you.

The following is a list of gifts that come from the seven chakras:

- The first or root chakra is unlimited intuition or gut feelings.

- The second or sexual chakra is sensing ideas, love, energies, and clairsentience through feeling nature and smells.

- The third or solar plexus is being sensitive to vibrations coming from other places or people.

- The fourth or heart chakra is having the ability to be empathetic with others since you have journeyed down the same path and you can see others going down. The thymus gives the gift of telepathy or the ability to communicate or speak to others with their mind.

- The fifth or throat chakra is clear hearing or hearing ideas and words on a higher vibrational level or sounds and music of the spiritual universe.

- The sixth or third eye chakra is clairvoyance or seeing clear. You will have the ability to see into the level that can't be seen with the eyes like seeing higher beings, energies, auras, and visions.

- The seventh or crown chakra is cosmic consciousness.

This chapter is a foundation that you can build your spiritual consciousness on. Each person will be at different place when they start. You can't begin a journey until you start one. You will need a roadmap to help you with where you are going. By understanding what makes up your energy fields, the chakras within our bodies, how they function, or don't function, and the disease that can occur by ignoring or repressing your feelings within our energetic system is a great start.

Everything we do in life is a choice. You need to always follow your inner guidance and voice.

This is a spiritual journey, and it doesn't matter what your religion. All of us are on a spiritual path, or we would not be on this planet. The tools for your transformation are given for your discernment and for you to use for your soul's best interest.

Conclusion

Thank for making it through to the end of *Chakra Healing For Beginners.* I hope it was informative and able to provide you with all of the tools you need to achieve your goals of creating more abundance in all the diverse areas of your life.

The next step is to start clearing your chakras. It's easy to start, and you will thank yourself later. Remember that whenever you have pain somewhere in your body, it can be traced back to your chakras. Go through the process and clear them one by one to remove any blockage. It may have to be done more than once and on a regular basis in order to get the most benefit.

We only have one body, one chance to make this minute matter. Make sure you live your life to the fullest and take care of yourself, so those around you will be able to be blessed, because you are in their lives. Life is full of opportunity. Take care of yourself. Those you love and who love you will be grateful to you for it.

Finally, if you found this book useful in any way, a positive review on Amazon is always appreciated!

Thanks again for buying my book.

I take reviews seriously and always look at them. This way, you are helping me provide you better content that you will LOVE in the future. A review doesn't have to be long, just one or two sentences and a number of stars you find appropriate (hopefully 5 of course).

Also, if I think your review is useful, I will mark it as "helpful." This will help you become more known on Amazon as a decent reviewer, and will ensure that more authors will contact you with free e-books in the future. This is how we can help each   other.

You can download any of my other books too. These are the titles:

NLP For Beginners

Parenting For Beginners

Here is an excerpt of another book I wrote, *NLP For Beginners: How To Create The Life You Want*

Introduction

First and foremost, I want to thank you for purchasing "*NLP for Beginners:* How to Create the Life You Want". This guidebook for beginners was created specifically with the intention of teaching you about a science constructed behind human behavior: Neuro-Linquistic Programming (NLP). You will learn about the NLP strategies that will best help you in creating the life you desire and transforming your dreams into a reality.

There are many people who believe that "the good life" is an illusion or story, similar to the "American Dream". These people believe that only individuals who are lucky or somehow picked due to random chance are the ones who are blessed with leading a life that represents their dreams. They believe that these luxurious and free lifestyles are a type of fortune that are not tangible or available to the average person, and therefore they cannot lead the life they desire. The reality is, anyone in the world has the ability to live "the good life". The good life is actually a life that is largely based on your own thoughts and the actions you take after having those thoughts.

Given this important information, we can conclude that absolutely anyone has the power to create and live their desired lifestyle. In order to do so, however, said person must first be willing to learn the necessary tools and practice integrating them into their own life.

If you have spent time dreaming about living the good life, but wondering how you would ever get there, then you are not unlike the majority of the people in this world. The most important thing to know is that this life is available to anyone who is willing to make it happen. All you need to do is will for it, and then implement the important tools you will learn in this book in order to bring your dream life into reality. It is as simple as asking for something, then taking necessary action to make it happen. In this case, you will be using NLP as your strategy to manifest your dream life and create the reality you want.

Up until now, everything you have ever wanted was simply a want, or a dream. If you are ready to start living a life where all of those dreams come to fruition and your reality is a mirror image of your desired life, then you are ready to start reading this book. Make sure you take your time and implement all of the strategies effectively, to ensure you get the most from this book and that your dream truly manifests into your reality.

Once again, thank you for purchasing this book, and best of luck in your journey.

Chapter 1: Change Your Thoughts

NLP is a tool that requires you to use your mind. Because of this, you need to be effective in controlling your own mind if you intend to control the minds of others. These strategies have many different terms, however the main component of them is to ensure that you are always in control of your own thoughts. This doesn't necessarily mean that you won't have negative or uncomfortable thoughts or feelings, simply that you will be able to control how you perceive them and what actions you take after experiencing them.

Essentially, before you use NLP on others, you need to know how to use it on yourself. To do this, there are various strategies of self-control you need to have in order to make it effective. In this chapter, we are going to explore the various steps you need to take in order to prepare your mind to create the reality you want in the outside world: beyond your imagination.

Recognize Your Thoughts

In order to control your thoughts, you must first recognize them. This can be difficult, as often we feel that our mind controls us, and not the other way around. While we don't always have control of what thoughts come to us, we can control how we perceive them, what we do after thinking them, and whether or not we allow ourselves to take action on those thoughts.

The best way to recognize your thoughts is to write them down in a thought journal. Usually, you will do this for about 48 hours. As you are writing down your thoughts, you will be actively recognizing them, while also practicing evaluating them. The goal is not to determine what thoughts are "bad" or "good", but merely to write them down, evaluate how they make you feel, and what you do as a result of experiencing those thoughts. The more you learn to recognize your thoughts through this physical practice, the easier it will be to recognize them as they come to you in the future. Once you start recognizing them, it is easier to control them and guide them in the direction you will for them to go.

Notice Thought Patterns

After you have taken a 48-hour account of your thoughts, you can analyze them to see what patterns you tend to have in your thoughts. You may notice that you feel particularly shy, weak or under confident in certain situations, while you feel strong, confident and courageous in others. This is completely normal. Ideally, you should have written down what circumstances you were in that caused each situation. If not, simply think back and take account. What sort of triggers do you notice are responsible for causing each level of thought pattern? How do these thought patterns serve you, if they do? Are you generally an optimist, or a pessimist? The more you are able to recognize your own thoughts and their patterns, the easier it will be to change them around so that you can develop the life you desire.

Flip Your Thoughts, Flip Your Life

This next step is going to be one of the most important steps you will take when it comes to successfully using NLP to change your life. You should ideally do this task on paper so that you can physically see and read the outcomes. You want to take your existing thoughts and flip them into the completely opposite direction. So, if you are thinking "I am not good enough" instead you should write down "I AM good enough". It is a simple switch, but it will have a very powerful effect on your mind. After writing down all of your switches, you will notice even more benefit if you actually say them out loud. You will get even more still from this practice if you say them out loud to yourself in front of a mirror, with total unwavering confidence in your voice, multiple times. This is called affirmations or incantations, and this practice is excellent in effectively helping you change your thought patterns.

Keep It Going

After you change your thought patterns on paper and say them out loud, you will want to make sure you continue on the path with changing your thoughts. It is not enough to simply say it once and then assume your entire life is changed. The reality is, it won't be. You need to consistently follow this pattern until it becomes a habit in your life. Recognize your thoughts, change them, and tell yourself the new thought. Repeat this until you no longer need to recognize the damaging thoughts because you immediately are able to take them and switch them around to be positive. Or, even better, they simply don't occur anymore. The more you complete this exercise, the easier this will become.

The Power of Positive Thinking: On Your Internal World

Positive thinking or positive beliefs are the basis for making virtually anything happen in your life. You may be surprised to know just how powerful positive thinking can be on your internal world. Positive thinking can have a significant impact on your health, joy, and overall quality of life. The more you practice positive thinking and implement positive thoughts where negative ones used to occur, the easier it will be for you to change your entire life.

According to well-known clinics, doctors, physicians, and other health care professionals, positive thinking has a greater effect on us than we may realize. When it comes to our own health specifically, positive thinking can actually make us healthier! There are many ways positive thinking enhances our quality of life, mentally and physically. Some include:

- Longer life
- Less risk of depression
- Less risk of stress or anxiety
- Greater resistance to common illnesses
- Healthier psychological and physical wellbeing
- Reduced risk of cardiovascular disease causing death
- Better coping skills

While it is unclear as to why exactly positive thinking can have such a strong impact on our health, doctors assume it is because those who are chronically optimistic are more likely to cope with stressful situations better. This ultimately causes them to avoid the added stress that worry, fear, and anxiety can cause. While it can be hard to become an optimist if you are used to being pessimistic, it is definitely doable and can be done with your perseverance and will.

The Power of Positive Thinking: On Your Reality

On your reality, positive thinking has many benefits that you simply can't deny. Those who are chronically optimistic tend to have lives that are more fulfilled. They are more likely to take opportunities that lead them to greater levels of success, they experience joy more deeply, and they are more enjoyable to be around. They tend to do well in almost anything they try, learn new skills easier, and adapt to life better. Because of these important abilities, they generally are capable of achieving anything they set their mind to, essentially turning their dreams into reality. Since this is exactly what you are trying to achieve, it is no wonder that having a positive mindset will have a great impact on your ability to take control of your life and lead the life you desire.

You may be aware of something called "The Law of Attraction". This law essentially states that you attract to you what you put out in the world. So, if you are consistently putting out positive intentions and are confident that, somehow, you will live your desired life, you will be much more likely to actually achieve it. While some believe this is solely a Law of the Universe, others conclude that it is because the more focused we are, the more likely we will take chances and opportunities that arise that can bring us closer to our dreams. Regardless of the specifics behind it, this law has been proven to work time and again. The more you practice positive thinking and attracting what you desire into life, the easier it will be to do so. This law, the Law of Attraction, is very important when it comes to NLP. In order for NLP to be successful, you will truly have to believe in your ability to make it work, as well as its ability to actually work. This belief will be one of the fundamental steps in mastering NLP and successfully changing your life.